NOURISH TO FLOURISH

The science of Female fertility and Nutrition

By

Dr. James Churchmann

TABLE OF CONTENTS

Introduction: Cultivating Fertility Through Nutrition

Chapter One: The Foundation of Female Fertility
1. The Miracle of Female Fertility
- Understanding the Gift of Life
2. Hormones and Fertility
- The Orchestra of Fertility
- The Role of Key Hormones

Chapter Two: Nutrient-Rich Eating for Fertility
3. The Nutrient Palette
- Essential Nutrients for Fertility
- Micronutrients and Their Role
4. Crafting a Fertility-Friendly Diet
- Building the Foundation of Nourishment
- Creating Balanced Meals

Chapter Three: Superfoods and Recipes for Fertility
5. Superfoods for Super Fertility
- Nutrient-Packed Powerhouses
- Integrating Superfoods into Your Diet
6. Wholesome Recipes for Nourishing Fertility
- Delightful Dishes for Fertility Wellness
- Cooking with Fertility in Mind

Chapter Four: Lifestyle and Fertility
7. The Impact of Lifestyle Choices on Fertility
- The Holistic Approach to Fertility
- Managing Stress and Its Role in Fertility
8. Mindful Living and Fertility

Conclusion

INTRODUCTION

Cultivating Fertility Through Nutrition

In the tapestry of life, few journeys are as remarkable and profound as the one that leads to motherhood. For countless generations, women have woven the threads of their family's legacy, shaping the future with their love and care. Today, the science of female fertility and nutrition offers a profound opportunity to enrich this age-old journey.

Welcome to "Nourish to Flourish: The Science of Female Fertility and Nutrition." Within these pages, we embark on a voyage of discovery, uncovering the delicate yet potent connection between the nourishment we provide our bodies and the flourishing of fertility. It's a journey that delves into the wonders of the female reproductive system, the intricate dance of hormones, and the remarkable power of nutrients to enhance our fertility.

Why, you might wonder, is this journey so crucial, so profoundly important? It's because female fertility is a profound gift, a force of nature, a cornerstone of life's continuity. It's about embracing the potential to conceive, nurture, and guide the growth of a new life. It's about the dreams and hopes of families, and the bonds woven with the arrival of each new generation.

Through this book, we will explore the science behind fertility, but we'll also go further. We'll delve into the art of nourishment, understanding the nutrients that fuel fertility, and crafting a fertility-friendly diet that can truly make a difference. You'll discover superfoods that can supercharge your fertility and relish the delightful recipes that will not only delight your palate but also enrich your fertility.

It's not just about diet; it's also about the broader context of lifestyle choices and their impact on fertility. Stress management, mindful living, and physical health are essential components of the flourishing fertility journey.

Moreover, this book isn't confined to a particular stage of life. We'll explore fertility across a woman's lifespan, from adolescence to menopause, and address fertility challenges along the way. We'll navigate the intricacies of fertility treatments, understanding assisted reproductive technologies and integrating nutrition into the process.

As we prepare for pregnancy and beyond, we'll guide you through preconception nutrition, and the vital role of partner support in this shared journey. Real-life success stories will inspire you, offering a glimpse into the possibilities that lie ahead.

In this exploration, we're not merely delving into science; we're celebrating the awe-inspiring power of nourishment. We're honoring the legacy of generations past and shaping the legacy of generations to come. We're nurturing not just life but the very essence of life itself.

So, join us as we embark on this journey of "Nourish to Flourish." Whether you're considering motherhood, already on the path, or simply intrigued by the marvel of life's creation, this book holds the key to understanding the science and art of female fertility and nutrition.

Your journey to nourishing to flourish begins here. It's a journey of wonder, empowerment, and possibility. Let's dive into the world of fertility and nourishment, where science and life's grand tapestry intersect.

The voyage is about to commence. Bon voyage!

As you embark on this profound journey, consider the incredible potential it holds. Within these pages, you'll gain a deeper understanding of your body's intricate mechanisms and how the choices you make, from the foods you select to the lifestyle you lead, can significantly impact your fertility.

Our exploration goes beyond the biological realm. It extends to the emotional and spiritual aspects of this journey. It's about harnessing not only the science of fertility but also the art of flourishing. It's about embracing the dreams and aspirations that come with the prospect of parenthood.

The modern world has provided us with unprecedented access to knowledge, and the science of fertility is no exception. Yet, amidst this wealth of information, there's often confusion. What's the right diet? How does stress affect fertility? What are the best practices for nourishing your body and soul on this journey?

This book is your guide, your companion on the path to flourishing fertility. It distills the complexities of science and the wisdom of nurturing into a readable, practical, and insightful resource. It is a place where research meets real-life experience, where expert advice is balanced with relatable stories. Your journey through "Nourish to Flourish" will equip you with the knowledge and tools to embark on this path of discovery with confidence. It will provide you with inspiration and insights to make informed choices about your diet, lifestyle, and overall well-being, tailored to your unique fertility journey.

So, whether you're standing at the threshold of motherhood, facing fertility challenges, or supporting someone on this journey, know that this book is here to accompany you. It's here to celebrate your individual story, to empower your choices, and to shine a light on the remarkable science and art of female fertility and nutrition.

Are you ready to embark on this journey of nourishment and flourishing fertility? The voyage is about to commence, and you're at the helm. Let the pages of "Nourish to Flourish" be your guide as you explore the boundless potential of female fertility and nutrition.

The journey is an extraordinary one, a journey of nurturing, empowerment, and life itself. It's a journey where science and soul intertwine, and your story is an integral part of this epic narrative. Welcome to "Nourish to Flourish." Your adventure begins now.

CHAPTER ONE
The Foundation of Female Fertility

Female fertility, the bedrock of human reproduction, is an intricate and finely tuned system. At its core, this foundation is built upon the cyclical interplay of hormones, the maturation of eggs, and the preparation of the uterus. Understanding the basics of this foundation is key to appreciating the miraculous journey of conception and childbirth. Join us as we explore the essential elements that underpin the marvel of female fertility.

1.The Miracle of Female Fertility

The miracle of female fertility is the extraordinary biological capability of a woman's body to conceive, nurture, and bring forth new life. This remarkable process showcases the intricacy and resilience of the female reproductive system, enabling the continuation of the human species and fostering a deep emotional and physical bond between mother and child. Female fertility is a testament to the wonders of nature and the potential for the creation of life

Here are 10 remarkable points that highlight the miracle of female fertility.

a. **The Menstrual Marvel:** Female fertility begins with the menstrual cycle, a precise and regulated process where hormones orchestrate the shedding of the uterine lining and the preparation for potential pregnancy.

b. **Ovulation's Precision:** Ovulation is a pivotal moment in the menstrual cycle when a mature egg is released from the ovary. This process is so finely tuned that it occurs like clockwork, typically in the middle of the cycle.

c. **Fertilization's Magic:** When sperm meets egg during fertilization, a zygote is formed, holding the potential for an entire human life. The fact that this tiny entity contains all the genetic information needed for a person is nothing short of miraculous.

d. **Implantation Artistry:** The fertilized egg journeys to the uterus and implants itself into the uterine lining. The female body's ability to recognize and support this new life is a remarkable feat.

e. **The Uterine Symphony:** As pregnancy progresses, the uterus undergoes astounding changes to accommodate the growing fetus. The transformation of the womb creates a secure environment for the baby.

f. **A Mother's Strength:** The culmination of female fertility is labor and childbirth, where the female body orchestrates the complex process of contractions, cervical dilation, and the safe delivery of the newborn. It's a testament to a mother's resilience and strength.

g. **Emotional Bonds:** Beyond the biological aspects, the emotional and psychological bond between a mother and her child is a unique and beautiful dimension of female fertility. It is through this connection that the nurturing and love for the child are expressed.

h. **Natural Family Planning:** Female fertility gives women the ability to decide when to start a family. Methods like natural family planning empower women to take charge of their reproductive choices.

i. **Support for Reproductive Health:** Recognizing the significance of female fertility highlights the importance of supporting women in their reproductive health, ensuring that they have the best chances for a healthy and successful pregnancy.

j. **A Continuation of Life's Story:** Female fertility is not just about the creation of individual lives but also about the continuation of the human story. It connects generations and perpetuates the legacy of humanity.

Female fertility is undeniably a miracle in every sense of the word. It showcases the intricate and harmonious processes that allow new life to come into the world. Understanding and celebrating this miracle emphasizes the importance of supporting and respecting the reproductive health of women and cherishing the awe-inspiring potential for new life that exists within every woman.

- **Understanding the Gift of Life**

Life, with all its complexity and beauty, is an extraordinary gift, and one of its most miraculous facets is the gift of female fertility. Let's explore how understanding the gift of life is intertwined with the awe-inspiring miracle of female fertility.

a. **The Beginning of Life:** Female fertility plays a pivotal role in the initiation of life. It's the bridge between the potential for existence and the actual creation of a new being. This process showcases the profound journey life takes from conception to birth.

b. **Creation and Nurture:** Female fertility is responsible for the creation of life, but it doesn't stop there. It includes the nurturing of life within the womb. The female body provides the ideal conditions for a developing embryo, illustrating the inherent value of each life.

c. **The Dance of Biology:** Female fertility involves the intricate dance of hormones, egg release, fertilization, and the formation of a zygote. Understanding this process helps us grasp the intricate biological mechanisms that underpin the creation of life.

d. **The Gift of Motherhood:** Female fertility culminates in motherhood, which is a profound and transformative experience. This journey includes not just the physical aspects but also the emotional and psychological connections that form between a mother and her child.

e. **Life's Precious Continuation:** Female fertility isn't just about individual lives; it's about the continuation of the human story. Recognizing this helps us appreciate the interconnectedness of generations and the legacy that fertility bestows upon humanity.

f. **Empowerment and Choice:** Understanding female fertility also involves recognizing a woman's autonomy over her reproductive choices. The ability to decide when and how to nurture life is a powerful aspect of this gift.

g. **Cherishing Life's Moments:** Embracing the gift of life includes cherishing moments of growth, from the inception of a new life within a woman's body to the first breath of a newborn. These moments are reminders of life's preciousness.

h. **Respecting Life's Vulnerability:** Female fertility emphasizes the vulnerability of life, especially during its early stages. Understanding this fragility encourages us to treat life with care and respect, from the moment of conception.

i. **The Power of Support:** In understanding female fertility, we acknowledge the importance of support systems, both medically and socially. Supporting women in their reproductive health ensures the continued miracle of life.

j. **Gratitude and Reverence:** The miracle of female fertility teaches us to approach life with gratitude and reverence. It highlights the importance of respecting and celebrating the potential for new life that exists within women.

In conclusion, understanding the gift of life is intricately tied to the miracle of female fertility. It invites us to marvel at the creation of life, embrace the journey from conception to birth, and acknowledge the profound impact it has on society and the world. Female fertility is a reminder of the beauty and wonder that life offers, a gift to be cherished, respected, and celebrated.

2. Hormones and Fertility

Hormones are the chemical messengers of the body, orchestrating a symphony of physiological processes, and among their many roles, they play a pivotal role in fertility. Understanding the intricate relationship between hormones and fertility is key to appreciating the complexity and beauty of the human reproductive system. These tiny molecules wield incredible power, governing the timing of ovulation, the preparation of the uterine lining for potential pregnancy, and the regulation of menstrual cycles. Join us in this exploration of how hormones are the silent conductors behind the miracle of fertility.

- **The Orchestra of Fertility: A Symphony of Life**

Fertility, the miraculous ability to bring new life into the world, is a symphony orchestrated by an ensemble of hormones, organs, and biological processes. Just as a conductor directs an orchestra, the female body conducts an intricate and harmonious performance to create life. In this exploration, we'll delve into the mesmerizing world of the "Orchestra of Fertility."

Act 1: Hormonal Prelude

The overture to this symphony is orchestrated by hormones. The pituitary gland secretes follicle-stimulating hormone (FSH), prompting the ovaries to begin the maturation of eggs. Meanwhile, luteinizing hormone (LH) prepares for the grand moment of ovulation. This hormonal prelude sets the stage for the main event.

Act 2: The Crescendo of Ovulation

As the curtains rise, the soloist, the ovary, takes the spotlight. With the precise timing of a seasoned musician, it releases a mature egg during ovulation. This moment, marked by the surge of LH, is the climactic point of the performance.

Act 3: The Fertilization Waltz

The duet between egg and sperm begins. While the egg waits in the fallopian tube, patiently, the sperm races to meet it. This dance, set to the rhythm of nature, concludes with the miraculous fusion of genetic material and the formation of a zygote.

Act 4: The Uterine Transformation

As the zygote journeys to the uterus, the uterine lining undergoes a transformation, preparing a soft and nourishing cradle for potential life. The endometrium thickens, ready to embrace the embryo in its care.

Act 5: The Emotional Adagio

While hormones and organs continue their dance, emotions join the symphony. The profound connection between a mother and her child is a heartfelt adagio. This emotional composition adds depth and meaning to the performance, encompassing love, anticipation, and dreams for the future.

Act 6: The Grand Finale

Finally, the grand finale, childbirth, is the culmination of this awe-inspiring symphony. The contractions of the uterus, the opening of the cervix, and the birth of a new life – it's an emotional and physical masterpiece that leaves the audience in wonder.

Curtain Call: Reflection and Legacy

As the orchestra takes its final bow, it leaves behind the legacy of life. Every performance contributes to the tapestry of humanity, and the music plays on as new generations take the stage.

The "Orchestra of Fertility" is a captivating masterpiece, where hormones, organs, and emotions converge to create life. It reminds us of the incredible intricacies of the human body and the profound significance of each new beginning. This symphony, with its cycles of hope, patience, and love, is a testament to the enduring miracle of fertility and the beauty of existence.

- **The Role of Key Hormones**

In the intricate tapestry of female fertility and reproduction, key hormones emerge as the virtuosos, orchestrating a symphony of life. These remarkable chemical messengers, secreted by glands and organs within the female body, guide the journey from puberty to motherhood. Join us on a captivating journey as we unveil the essential roles played by these hormone virtuosos in the realm of female fertility and reproduction.

Act 1: Follicle-Stimulating Hormone (FSH)

FSH takes center stage as the overture to the performance. This hormone, released by the pituitary gland, triggers the development of ovarian follicles. These tiny sacs cradle immature eggs, setting the scene for the ovulatory process.

Act 2: Luteinizing Hormone (LH)

As the symphony builds, LH enters with a resounding crescendo. Its surge, also orchestrated by the pituitary gland, is responsible for triggering ovulation. The matured egg is released from the ovary, poised to meet its counterpart for fertilization.

Act 3: Estrogen

Estrogen takes the stage with grace and elegance. Primarily produced by the ovaries, it exerts influence throughout the female body. Estrogen governs the menstrual cycle, ensuring that the uterine lining thickens, ready to receive a fertilized egg. It's also responsible for secondary sexual characteristics and plays a central role in the health of the reproductive system.

Act 4: Progesterone

With a nurturing presence, progesterone follows estrogen. Produced by the corpus luteum in the ovary, this hormone sustains the uterine lining. If fertilization occurs, it creates the perfect environment for the embryo to implant and grow. It's the embodiment of maternal preparation.

Act 5: Human Chorionic Gonadotropin (hCG)

In the enchanting moment of conception, HCG takes the spotlight. This hormone, produced by the placenta, declares the onset of pregnancy. It sustains the corpus luteum, ensuring a supportive and nourishing environment for the embryo.

Act 6: Prolactin and Oxytocin

Prolactin and oxytocin enter with a sense of nurturing. Prolactin, secreted by the pituitary gland, stimulates milk production in the mammary glands, enabling the nurturing of an infant. Oxytocin, often referred to as the "love hormone," triggers milk ejection and uterine contractions during childbirth, fostering the emotional bond between mother and child.

As the symphony concludes, it leaves behind the legacy of human life. These virtuoso hormones extend their roles far beyond mere biology. They influence not only the physical aspects of reproduction but also the emotional and nurturing bonds that define the human experience.

The virtuoso hormones in the realm of female fertility and reproduction are true maestros of life's symphony. From orchestrating fertility and sustaining pregnancy to nurturing newborns, they are the conductors of a complex, intricate, and breathtaking performance. The harmony and balance they bring to the journey from womanhood to motherhood are nothing short of miraculous, celebrating the profound beauty of the female reproductive system.

CHAPTER TWO
Nutrient-Rich Eating for Fertility

In the grand tapestry of life, the quest for fertility is a powerful and deeply human desire. Nutrient-rich eating stands as a cornerstone in this journey, offering the promise of optimizing reproductive health. This is more than a dietary approach; it's a profound step toward enhancing the potential for new life. In this introduction, we begin our exploration of nutrient-rich eating for female fertility, a path that blends science, nature, and the art of nourishing the body.

A. The Fertility Journey: A Universal Desire

The desire to conceive and nurture new life is one of the most fundamental human aspirations. For countless generations, women have sought the secrets to this magical journey. Today, science and nutrition unveil a path toward enhancing the odds of conception and the promise of a healthy pregnancy.

B. Nutrient-Rich Eating: The Foundation of Fertility

At its core, nutrient-rich eating is about providing the body with the essential elements it needs to function optimally. For women seeking fertility, this dietary approach is a means of harmonizing the intricate processes within the reproductive system. From the quality of eggs to the hormonal balance, nutrients serve as the building blocks of life.

C. The Power of Nutrients

Vitamins, minerals, proteins, and other nutrients are not just scientific terms but vital players in the fertility symphony. Folate prevents birth defects; omega-3 fatty acids regulate hormones; antioxidants protect precious eggs and sperm. Each nutrient has a role to play in the intricate choreography of reproduction.

D. Beyond Food: A Holistic Approach

Yet, the journey to fertility goes beyond what's on your plate. Stress management, physical activity, and emotional well-being all contribute to a holistic approach. The mind-body connection becomes a powerful ally in the quest for conception.

E. A Nourishing Journey Begins

As we embark on this journey into the heart of nutrient-rich eating for female fertility, we embrace the opportunity to empower women with knowledge and tools to optimize their reproductive health. It's a celebration of life's greatest miracle, an ode to new beginnings, and a profound step toward nurturing the next generation. Join us as we delve deeper into the art and science of nourishing life, one nutrient at a time.

3. The Nutrient Palette

In the delicate realm of female fertility, the nutrient palate is akin to a vibrant artist's palette, each nutrient representing a unique color that contributes to the masterpiece of reproductive health. Just as an artist carefully selects their hues to create a stunning work of art, women can harness the power of nutrients to optimize their fertility journey. This introduction opens the door to an exploration of how these essential elements blend together to paint a beautiful picture of fertility.

A. The Palette of Life

Imagine the human body as a canvas, and every nutrient as a distinct color, essential to creating life's most intricate and beautiful artwork. This palette, rich with vitamins, minerals, proteins, and more, provides the foundation for reproductive health.

B. Folate: The Blueprint of Life

Folate, a vital nutrient, is the equivalent of the blueprint that guides a construction project. It ensures that the development of a new life begins with a sturdy foundation, preventing birth defects and fostering a healthy start.

C. Omega-3 Fatty Acids: The Regulators of Hormones

Omega-3 fatty acids, the gentle strokes of regulation, keep the hormonal balance in check. These essential fats, like skilled conductors, ensure that the reproductive system functions harmoniously.

E. Antioxidants: The Guardians of Vitality Antioxidants stand as the protectors of life's vitality, shielding eggs and sperm from the ravages of oxidative stress. Like a fortress, they safeguard the integrity of the genetic material.

F. Nutrients as Artists: Just as artists meticulously create their works, each nutrient plays its part. From proteins that provide the building blocks for hormones to vitamins and minerals that serve as essential tools in this intricate creation, the nutrient palate is a diverse and nuanced array.

G. **Creating Life's Masterpiece:** In the pages that follow, we will explore the role of each nutrient as they contribute to the grand composition of female fertility. This journey is a celebration of life's most remarkable art form – the creation of new life – and an invitation to savor the beauty and complexity of the nutrient palate. Join us as we unveil the artistry of nourishing life, brushstroke by brushstroke, nutrient by nutrient.

- **Essential Nutrients for Fertility**

In the captivating world of female fertility, essential nutrients act as the building blocks of life. These powerful elements serve as the foundation upon which the delicate journey of conception, pregnancy, and motherhood is constructed. Join us in this exploration as we uncover the remarkable role of these nutrients, nourishing the path to fertility and the creation of new life.

A. **Folate (Vitamin B9):** Folate is crucial for the development of the neural tube in a developing fetus, preventing birth defects like spina bifida. It's essential for early pregnancy when the neural tube forms.

Sources: Leafy greens, citrus fruits, beans, and fortified cereals.

B. **Omega-3 Fatty Acids:** Omega-3s help regulate hormones, reduce inflammation, and improve the quality of cervical mucus, which is vital for sperm transport.

Sources: Fatty fish like salmon and mackerel, flaxseeds, chia seeds, and walnuts.

C. **Antioxidants (Vitamins C & E, Selenium, Zinc):** Antioxidants protect eggs and sperm from oxidative stress, reducing the risk of DNA damage and improving overall reproductive health.

Sources: Citrus fruits, nuts, seeds, and lean meat for zinc; sunflower seeds and almonds for vitamin E; and Brazil nuts for selenium.

D. **Protein**: Amino acids from protein sources are the building blocks for hormones that control the menstrual cycle and ovulation. They also support overall reproductive health.

Sources: Lean meats, poultry, fish, beans, lentils, and dairy products.

E. **Vitamins and Minerals (Vitamin D, Iron, Calcium):** These nutrients play various roles in fertility, including hormone regulation, egg quality, and maintaining a healthy uterus.

Sources: Sun exposure for vitamin D; lean red meat, leafy greens, and fortified cereals for iron; and dairy products for calcium.

F. **Plant-Based Nutrition:** Plant-based diets rich in fruits, vegetables, whole grains, and plant-based proteins have been associated with improved fertility. They provide a large number of essential nutrients.

Sources: Include a variety of fruits, vegetables, whole grains, legumes (lentils, chickpeas), nuts, and seeds in your diet.

It's important to maintain a balanced and diverse diet to ensure you receive these essential nutrients. A well-rounded diet supports overall health, including reproductive health. Additionally, consider consulting a healthcare professional or nutritionist for personalized guidance on nutrition and fertility.

- **Micronutrients and Their Roles in Female Fertility**

Micronutrients, which include vitamins and minerals, are the unsung heroes of female fertility. While they are required in smaller quantities compared to macronutrients like proteins and carbohydrates, their roles in maintaining reproductive health are immense. These tiny compounds play a vital part in supporting the various stages of the female reproductive journey.

A. **Folate (Vitamin B9):** Folate is paramount during the early stages of pregnancy. It prevents neural tube defects in the developing fetus, ensuring proper spinal cord and brain formation. It also supports the production of DNA and RNA.

Sources: Leafy greens, citrus fruits, beans, fortified cereals.

B. **Iron:** Iron is important for the transport of oxygen in the blood. In relation to fertility, adequate iron levels are vital for healthy ovulation and the development of a receptive uterine lining.

Sources: Lean red meat, beans, lentils, fortified cereals, spinach.

C. **Calcium:** Calcium is necessary for uterine muscle function and cell communication. It supports the health of the female reproductive system, including the regulation of the menstrual cycle.

Sources: Dairy products, fortified plant-based milks, broccoli, almonds.

D. **Vitamin D:** Vitamin D helps regulate hormones and supports the immune system. It may play a role in improving the chances of conceiving, although more research is needed in this area.

Sources: Sunlight, fatty fish (e.g., salmon), fortified dairy products.

E. **Vitamin E:** Vitamin E is an antioxidant that helps protect cells, including reproductive cells, from oxidative stress. It contributes to egg and sperm health.

Sources: Nuts (e.g., almonds), seeds (e.g., sunflower seeds), spinach.

F. **Selenium:** Selenium is another antioxidant that helps protect the ovaries and sperm from oxidative damage. It supports optimal reproductive function.

Sources: Brazil nuts, fish, turkey.

G. **Zinc:** Zinc is essential for the production of mature eggs and the maintenance of a healthy menstrual cycle. It also plays a role in embryo development.

Sources: Lean meat, dairy products, nuts, beans.

H. **Omega-3 Fatty Acids:** Omega-3s help regulate hormones, reduce inflammation, and improve the quality of cervical mucus. This enhances the environment for sperm to reach the egg.

Sources: Fatty fish (e.g., salmon), flaxseeds, chia seeds.

I. **B Vitamins (B6, B12):** B vitamins, particularly B6 and B12, play a role in hormone regulation and ovulation. They also support overall reproductive health.

Sources: Poultry, fish, fortified cereals, dairy products.

These micronutrients are essential for the intricate dance of hormones, ovulation, and the nurturing of a potential pregnancy. A well-balanced diet that includes a variety of nutrient-rich foods ensures that your body has the necessary micronutrients to support female fertility. If you are planning to conceive or facing fertility challenges, consulting a healthcare provider or nutritionist can provide personalized guidance to optimize your nutrient intake.

4. Crafting a Fertility-Friendly Diet

The journey to parenthood begins long before conception. Crafting a fertility-friendly diet is a powerful and proactive step towards optimizing your reproductive health. This introduction sets the stage for exploring the art of nourishing your body to enhance fertility, covering the key principles, nutrient-rich choices, and lifestyle factors that contribute to the creation of a welcoming environment for new life.

Conception is not a sudden event but the culmination of factors that lead to a fertile ground. A fertility-friendly diet isn't just about what you eat; it's about preparing your body for the miraculous journey ahead.

- **Understanding the Science of Fertility**

It's essential to comprehend the intricate science of fertility, from ovulation to the role of hormones. This knowledge provides the backdrop for making informed dietary choices.

The Principles of Fertility-Friendly Eating

a. *Balancing Nutrients:* Ensuring a well-rounded intake of essential nutrients, including vitamins, minerals, and macronutrients like proteins and healthy fats.

b. *Antioxidant Rich:* Embracing foods that are rich in antioxidants to protect reproductive cells from oxidative stress.

c. *Hormone Regulation:* Incorporating foods that help regulate hormones, such as omega-3 fatty acids.

d. *Weight and Fertility:* Addressing the connection between weight and reproductive health to find a healthy balance.

e. *Nutrient-Packed Foods*: This guide will delve into the foods that serve as the nutrient-packed heroes of a fertility-friendly diet. From leafy greens and lean proteins to fertility superfoods, we'll explore how these elements support reproductive health.

f. *Plant-Based Power:* Discover the advantages of plant-based nutrition for fertility. A diet rich in fruits, vegetables, whole grains, and plant-based proteins offers a plethora of nutrients that support fertility.

g. *A Holistic Approach:* Beyond what's on your plate, we'll explore the importance of managing stress, staying active, and maintaining emotional well-being. These aspects are crucial for crafting a holistic approach to fertility.

h. *Consulting the Experts:* While this guide provides a foundation for crafting a fertility-friendly diet, it's always wise to seek professional guidance. Healthcare providers and nutritionists can offer personalized recommendations to optimize your fertility journey.

A fertility-friendly diet is not a destination but a nurturing journey. It's an embrace of life's greatest miracle and an ode to new beginnings. Join us as we uncover the art and science of nourishing life, step by step, choice by choice, as you craft a fertility-friendly diet to prepare your body for the journey of parenthood.

- **Building the Foundation of Nourishment:** *The Cornerstone of Health and Wellness*

In the grand tapestry of life, nourishment stands as the cornerstone upon which our health, well-being, and vitality are built. Just as a sturdy foundation supports the most magnificent structures, the quality of nourishment we provide our bodies underpins our physical, mental, and emotional health. This exploration takes us on a journey to understand the profound importance of building a strong foundation of nourishment and its transformative impact on our lives.

a. **The Foundation of Health:** Before any great edifice can rise, there must be a foundation that can withstand the test of time. In our lives, this foundation is health, and at its core is nourishment. Nourishment not only sustains us but also fuels our potential for growth and well-being.

b. **Understanding the Power of Nourishment:** It's essential to comprehend the science and significance of nourishment. The macronutrients (proteins, fats, and carbohydrates) and micronutrients (vitamins and minerals) serve as the building blocks of life, influencing every aspect of our existence.

c. **Building Blocks of Nourishment**

Macronutrients: The sources of energy, repair, and growth in our bodies, they include proteins, which build and repair tissues, carbohydrates, which provide energy, and fats, which are crucial for cell health.

Micronutrients: These vitamins and minerals, although required in smaller quantities, play vital roles in metabolism, immunity, and overall health.

Antioxidants: These compounds protect our cells from oxidative stress, helping to maintain health and prevent chronic diseases.

Hydration: The often underestimated foundation of health, water is essential for every bodily function.

d. The Impact on Well-Being: The quality of our nourishment has a profound impact on our overall well-being. It influences our energy levels, mental clarity, emotional balance, and physical resilience.

e. The Role of Whole Foods: Whole, unprocessed foods are the bedrock of a nourishing foundation. They provide a plethora of essential nutrients and fiber, supporting both physical and mental health.

f. Beyond the Plate: A Holistic Approach

While nourishment is a pivotal part of our foundation, a holistic approach to well-being encompasses more. Physical activity, stress management, and emotional well-being are equally significant components that shape our health and happiness.

g. Seeking Guidance: Navigating the path to building a strong foundation of nourishment may require professional guidance. Healthcare providers and nutritionists offer personalized support and recommendations.

h. The Journey to Wholeness: The construction of a strong foundation of nourishment is a journey to wholeness. It's a celebration of life's most precious gift—the gift of health. Join us as we explore the art and science of nourishing life, one choice at a time, to build the foundation of wellness, vitality, and a flourishing future

- **Creating Balance Meals**

Balanced meals are the cornerstone of good health and fertility. They provide not only nourishment but also the energy and nutrients necessary to support the intricate processes of the reproductive system. This exploration dives into the art of crafting balanced meals that can enhance your fertility and overall well-being, ensuring your body is primed for the journey to parenthood.

A. The Harmony of Balanced Meals

Just as a symphony relies on the interplay of various instruments to create beautiful music, our bodies depend on the harmonious combination of nutrients to function optimally. Balanced meals are the arrangement of these nutrients in a way that sustains and nurtures our physical and emotional health.

B. Understanding the Components of Balance

Balanced meals are built upon key components, each with a specific role:

Proteins: Provide the building blocks for hormones and tissues. Essential for ovarian health, menstrual cycle regulation, and fertility.

Carbohydrates: Carbohydrates support regular menstrual cycles and hormone balance.

Fats: Crucial for hormone production, especially the fertility-regulating hormones. They also help the body absorb fat-soluble vitamins.

Fiber: Aids in digestion, regulates blood sugar levels, and supports overall health.

Vitamins and Minerals: Play a role in hormone balance, ovulation, and the health of reproductive organs.

C. Building Balanced Meals for Fertility

Proteins: Lean meats, poultry, fish, eggs, legumes (e.g., beans, lentils), and dairy products.
Carbohydrates: Whole grains (e.g., quinoa, brown rice), fruits, and vegetables.
Fats: Nuts, seeds, avocados, and olive oil.
Fiber: Whole grains, fruits, vegetables, and legumes.

Vitamins and Minerals: A diverse array of colorful fruits and vegetables, leafy greens, and fortified foods.

D. The Role of Whole Foods

Whole, unprocessed foods are at the heart of balanced meals. They provide a rich array of nutrients, fiber, and antioxidants that support fertility and overall well-being.

E. Meal Planning for Fertility

Begin with a protein source, such as lean meat, beans, or fish.
Add a variety of colorful vegetables and fruits for essential vitamins and minerals.
Incorporate whole grains for carbohydrates and fiber.
Include healthy fats, like avocados or nuts, in moderation.
Stay hydrated with water and herbal teas.

Balance in fertility also involves stress management, physical activity, and emotional well-being. A holistic approach is essential to support both fertility and overall health.

Crafting balanced meals is not only a path to fertility but a journey to optimal health. It's about embracing the gift of life and celebrating the profound beauty of well-being. Join us as we delve into the art and science of nourishing life, one balanced meal at a time, to create the harmonious symphony of fertility and wellness

CHAPTER THREE
Superfoods and Recipes for Super Fertility

5. Superfood for Super Fertility

In the pursuit of parenthood, nutrition can be a powerful ally. Superfoods, brimming with vital nutrients and antioxidants, offer a concise yet profound strategy to enhance fertility. This brief introduction opens the door to the world of superfoods and their extraordinary potential in the journey to conception.

- **Nutrient-Packed Powerhouses: Enhancing Female Fertility**

In the intricate dance of female fertility, the significance of nutrition cannot be understated. Nutrient-packed powerhouses emerge as the unsung heroes, delivering the essential elements that harmonize the delicate processes of conception and reproduction. This exploration delves into the vital role of these nutritional champions and their profound impact on female fertility.

a. **The Quest for Fertility:** The journey toward motherhood is a profound aspiration shared by women across the world. Nutrient-packed powerhouses provide the fuel for this remarkable journey, enriching the foundation upon which new life can flourish.

b. **Understanding the Power of Nutrition:** Nutrition is not merely about sustenance; it is the art of nourishing the body to its fullest potential. In the realm of fertility, this means providing the body with the precise nutrients required to optimize the environment for conception

c. **Nutrient-Packed Powerhouses: The Unsung Heroes:** These nutritional champions are not just foods; they are extraordinary reservoirs of vitamins, minerals, antioxidants, and other essential elements. They are the secret ingredients that influence the quality of eggs, the regulation of hormones, and the overall health of the reproductive system.

d. **Exploring the Nutrient-Packed Powerhouses**

Berries: Bursting with antioxidants, they shield reproductive cells from oxidative stress.
Leafy Greens: Abundant in folate and other vital nutrients, they support a healthy pregnancy.
Fatty Fish: Rich in omega-3 fatty acids, they regulate hormones and improve egg quality.
Nuts and Seeds: Provide a balance of healthy fats and protein, nurturing reproductive health.
Legumes: High in plant-based nutrients, they enhance fertility and support overall well-being.

e. **Beyond Nutrition:** while nutrient-packed powerhouses are crucial, the fertility journey extends beyond the dinner plate. Managing stress, staying physically active, and fostering emotional well-being create a holistic approach that enhances the chances of conception.

f. **Consulting the Guides of Fertility:** In the realm of fertility, seeking guidance from healthcare providers and nutritionists provides the knowledge and support necessary to personalize your nutritional approach for enhanced reproductive health.

Nutrient-packed powerhouses are the choreographers of fertility, the unsung heroes that add grace and strength to the dance of conception. They are your allies in the pursuit of motherhood, the champions of a healthy and vibrant reproductive journey. Join us as we explore the art and science of nourishing life, one nutrient-packed powerhouse at a time, to empower the incredible dance of female fertility.

- **Integrating Superfoods into Your Diet**

Superfoods, nature's nutritional powerhouses, are a simple yet profound way to elevate your diet. These foods are packed with essential nutrients and antioxidants that can have a positive impact on your health. Incorporating them into your daily meals doesn't require a major overhaul of your eating habits. Here's a concise guide to integrating superfoods into your diet:

a. **Start with One Superfood:** Begin by selecting one superfood that appeals to you. It could be something readily available in your region or something you already enjoy.

b. **Incorporate Superfoods Gradually:** Instead of completely replacing your existing foods, add superfoods to your current meals. For instance, top your morning yogurt with berries or sprinkle chia seeds on your salad.

c. **Mix and Match**: Superfoods can complement each other. Consider creating a smoothie with a mix of berries, spinach, and a dash of flaxseeds.

d. **Snack on Superfoods:** Swap out processed snacks for superfood snacks. Instead of chips, munch on a handful of nuts or a small serving of dark chocolate (with a high cocoa content).

e. **Experiment with Superfood Recipes:** Explore recipes that incorporate superfoods. Try a quinoa salad with colorful veggies, or make a salmon dish seasoned with herbs and spices.

f. **Plan Balanced Meals:** Superfoods can be part of balanced meals. Build a plate that includes lean protein, whole grains, and plenty of colorful vegetables, and add superfoods as a side or garnish.

g. **Stay Consistent:** Regularity is key. Keep superfoods in your diet over time, making them a natural part of your eating routine.

h. **Be Mindful of Portions:** Superfoods are nutrient-dense, so you don't need large quantities. A little goes a long way.

i. **Stay Hydrated:** Don't forget the importance of water. Superfoods can be dehydrating, so ensure you maintain a proper water intake.

j. **Enjoy the Process:** Eating should be pleasurable. Choose superfoods that you genuinely enjoy, and savor the experience.

Incorporating superfoods into your diet is a step toward a healthier and more vibrant lifestyle. Over time, you'll find that these nutrient-rich additions not only enhance your well-being but also contribute to the delicious diversity of your meals.

6. Wholesome Recipes for Nourishing Fertility

The path to parenthood is a remarkable journey, and a well-balanced diet can be a vital companion on this quest. Here, we present three wholesome recipes designed to nourish fertility by incorporating nutrient-dense ingredients that support reproductive health.

A. Fertility-Boosting Smoothie:

Ingredients:

- 1 cup of mixed berries (strawberries, blueberries, raspberries)
- 1 ripe banana
- 1 cup spinach or kale
- 1 tablespoon flaxseeds
- 1/2 cup Greek yogurt
- 1 cup of almond milk (or your preferred milk)
- 1 tablespoon honey (optional)

Instructions:

1. Add the mixed berries, banana, spinach or kale, flaxseeds, Greek yogurt, and almond milk to a blender.
2. Blend until smooth and creamy.
3. Taste and add honey for sweetness, if desired.

4. Pour into a glass and savor this nutrient-packed fertility booster. Enjoy it as a morning meal or a refreshing snack

B. Quinoa and Veggie Power Bowl:

Ingredients:

- 1 cup quinoa
- 2 cups water or vegetable broth
- 1 cup cherry tomatoes, halved
- 1 cup cucumber, diced
- 1/2 red bell pepper, diced
- 1/4 red onion, finely chopped
- 1/4 cup fresh parsley, chopped
- 1/4 cup crumbled feta cheese (optional)
- 2 tablespoons extra-virgin olive oil
- 1 tablespoon lemon juice
- Salt and pepper to taste

Instruction:

1. Rinse the quinoa with cold water and dry.
2. In a medium saucepan, bring 2 cups of water or vegetable broth to a boil. Add the quinoa, reduce heat, cover, and simmer for 15-20 minutes until the quinoa is cooked and the liquid is absorbed. Let it cool.
3. Combine or mix the cooked quinoa, cherry tomatoes, cucumber, red bell pepper, red onion, and parsley.
4. In a small bowl, whisk together the olive oil, lemon juice, salt, and pepper.
5. Drizzle the dressing over the quinoa and veggie mixture and toss gently to combine.

6. Top with crumbled feta cheese if desired.
7. This nutrient-rich power bowl makes for a delicious and wholesome lunch or dinner.

C. Baked Salmon with Lemon and Asparagus:

Ingredients:

- 2 salmon fillets
- 1 bunch of fresh asparagus
- 2 tablespoons olive oil
- 1 lemon, thinly sliced
- 2 cloves garlic, minced
- Salt and pepper to taste
- dill or parsley for garnish

Instructions:

1. Preheat your oven to 375°F (190°C).
2. Put the salmon filets on a baking sheet lined with parchment paper.
3. Arrange the asparagus spears around the salmon.
4. Drizzle olive oil over the salmon and asparagus.
5. Sprinkle minced garlic, salt, and pepper evenly over both the salmon and asparagus.
6. Lay lemon slices on top of the salmon.
7. Bake for 15-20 minutes, or until the salmon flakes easily with a fork and the asparagus is tender.
8. Garnish with fresh dill or parsley before serving.

These recipes are not just delicious but are also designed to enrich your diet with the nutrients essential for supporting fertility. However, remember that individual dietary needs may vary, so it's advisable to consult with a healthcare provider or nutritionist for personalized guidance on nutrition and fertility.

- **Delightful Dishes for Fertility Wellness**

Fertility wellness involves not only the nutrients you consume but also the enjoyment of what you eat. Here, we enumerate and explain a selection of delightful dishes that not only support fertility but also satisfy your taste buds.

A. Berry and Spinach Salad:

Ingredients:

- Fresh spinach leaves
- Mixed berries (strawberries, blueberries, raspberries)
- Chopped nuts (almonds, walnuts, or pecans)
- Feta cheese (optional)
- Balsamic vinaigrette dressing

Explanation:

This colorful salad is rich in fertility-friendly nutrients. Spinach provides folate, while mixed berries offer antioxidants and essential vitamins. Nuts add healthy fats and protein. The optional feta cheese provides a creamy touch. Top it with balsamic vinaigrette for a delightful and nutritious meal.

B. Grilled Salmon with Asparagus:

Ingredients:

- Fresh salmon fillets
- Fresh asparagus
- Olive oil
- Lemon juice
- Garlic
- Fresh herbs (dill or parsley)
- Salt and pepper

Explanation:

Salmon is a superb source of omega-3 fatty acids, which regulate hormones and improve egg quality. Asparagus provides folate and fiber. Season the dish with garlic, lemon, and fresh herbs for a delightful flavor that enhances fertility wellness.

C. Quinoa and Veggie Stir-Fry:

Ingredients:

- Quinoa
- Assorted colorful vegetables (bell peppers, broccoli, carrots)
- Tofu or lean chicken breast
- Low-sodium soy sauce or a stir-fry sauce of your choice
- Ginger and garlic
- Sesame seeds for garnish

Explanation:

Quinoa offers plant-based protein and fiber, supporting hormone balance. Colorful vegetables provide essential vitamins and minerals. Tofu or lean chicken adds extra protein. This stir-fry is seasoned with ginger, garlic, and soy sauce for a delectable and fertility-enhancing meal.

D. Greek Yogurt Parfait:

Ingredients:

- Greek yogurt
- Fresh mixed berries
- Honey or maple syrup
- Granola (optional)
- Chopped nuts (e.g., almonds or walnuts)

Explanation:

Greek yogurt is a protein-rich choice that supports reproductive health. Berries provide antioxidants and essential vitamins. Add a drizzle of honey, granola, and chopped nuts for a delightful parfait that not only nourishes but also satisfies your sweet cravings.

E. Sweet Potato and Chickpea Curry:

Ingredients:

- Sweet potatoes
- Chickpeas
- Spinach or kale
- Coconut milk
- Curry spices (turmeric, cumin, coriander)
- Garlic and ginger
- Basmati rice (optional)

Explanation:

Sweet potatoes are rich in beta-carotene, which may support fertility. Chickpeas add protein and fiber, while spinach or kale provides essential nutrients. The curry spices infuse this dish with delightful flavors, creating a nourishing and satisfying meal.

These delightful dishes not only cater to your taste buds but also cater to your fertility wellness. By enjoying these nutrient-rich and balanced meals, you can promote reproductive health while savoring the journey to parenthood.

- **Cooking with Fertility in Mind: Nourishing Your Path to Parenthood**

The kitchen is a place where magic happens, and it can be a hub for nurturing your fertility journey. Cooking with fertility in mind isn't just about delicious meals; it's about crafting dishes that support your reproductive health. In this culinary adventure, we explore how you can create a fertility-friendly kitchen and offer a range of delightful, nutritious recipes to inspire your path to parenthood.

Creating a Fertility-Friendly Kitchen

a. **Choose Nutrient-Packed Ingredients:** Select ingredients that are rich in fertility-boosting nutrients. Think fresh fruits, colorful vegetables, lean proteins, whole grains, and nutrient-dense superfoods.
b. **Incorporate Healthy Fats:** Healthy fats, such as avocados, nuts, and olive oil, are vital for hormone production and reproductive health.
c. **Opt for Plant-Based Proteins:** Consider plant-based proteins like beans, lentils, and tofu. They provide essential nutrients without the saturated fats found in some animal proteins.
d. **Embrace Whole Grains:** Whole grains like quinoa, brown rice, and oats are a superb source of fiber, which supports hormonal balance.
e. **Mindful Meat Choices:** If you consume meat, choose lean options and aim for organic or pasture-raised selections when possible.

By embracing these fertility-friendly kitchen strategies and savoring these delightful recipes, you're not only nourishing your body but also cultivating an environment that promotes fertility wellness. It's a culinary journey that can lead to the remarkable destination of parenthood, one wholesome and delicious meal at a time.

CHAPTER FOUR

Lifestyle and Fertility

7. The Impact of Lifestyle Choices on Fertility

In the intricate tapestry of life, the desire to create a family is a profound and universal aspiration. The journey to parenthood is marked by excitement, anticipation, and, for many, the question of when and how it will happen. In this exploration, we delve into a critical chapter of this journey – the profound impact of lifestyle choices on fertility.

a. **The Quest for Parenthood:** The desire to nurture and bring new life into the world is woven into the fabric of human existence. For countless generations, this quest has been a common thread connecting the past, present, and future.

b. **The Intricacies of Fertility:** Fertility is a delicate and complex orchestra of biological processes. It is the culmination of myriad factors working in harmony to bring forth the miracle of life. While biology plays a central role, our lifestyle choices have emerged as crucial actors on this stage.

c. **Lifestyle as the Pivot Point:** Our lifestyle choices, encompassing what we eat, how we exercise, our stress management, and even our social habits, all hold the potential to influence fertility profoundly. The decisions we make regarding our well-being today can shape our future family in ways both profound and lasting.

d. **Balancing Act: Nutrition, Physical Activity, and Emotional Well-Being**

The impact of lifestyle on fertility is a multifaceted story. The choices we make regarding our nutrition, level of physical activity, and emotional well-being collectively shape the terrain where fertility unfolds. A balanced diet rich in vital nutrients, a healthy approach to exercise, and strategies for managing stress are integral parts of this narrative.

e. Beyond Biology: Social and Environmental Considerations

It's not just what we do, but also the world we inhabit. Social, environmental, and occupational factors, from exposure to toxins to the support we receive from our communities, can all play a role in the story of fertility.

f. **The Need for Knowledge and Empowerment:** Understanding the impact of lifestyle choices on fertility is a voyage into knowledge, empowerment, and ultimately, conscious decision-making. By unraveling this complex web, we can equip ourselves with the information to make choices that are conducive to our aspirations.

g. **A Journey of Conscious Choices**

The pages ahead unveil the intricate ways in which lifestyle choices influence fertility. It is a journey of enlightenment, of appreciating the remarkable interplay of biology, environment, and conscious decisions. As we navigate the terrain of lifestyle and fertility, we set sail on a quest toward understanding, empowering, and ultimately, celebrating the wondrous journey to parenthood.

- **The Holistic Approach to Fertility: Nurturing Life's Most Profound Journey**

The desire to create life is a deeply human longing, shared across cultures, continents, and generations. The path to parenthood is a remarkable journey filled with hope, anticipation, and love. In this exploration, we embark on the profound journey of a holistic approach to fertility—a path that not only recognizes the biological aspects but also acknowledges the intricate interplay of mind, body, and spirit in the remarkable journey of conception.

a. **The Wholeness of Fertility:** Fertility is more than just the mechanics of egg and sperm. It is the holistic expression of life, reflecting our overall well-being and vitality. A holistic approach recognizes that fertility is not isolated from the rest of our existence; it is an integral part of our physical, emotional, and mental health.

b. **Nutrition: The Foundation of Fertility**

Nutrition forms the bedrock of fertility. What we eat is not only sustenance but the nourishment that fuels the complex processes of reproduction. A diet rich in vital nutrients, including antioxidants, healthy fats, and essential vitamins, creates an environment in which fertility can flourish.

c. **Physical Activity: The Dance of Well-Being**

Physical activity contributes to fertility in multifaceted ways. It regulates hormones, supports weight management, and enhances emotional well-being. A balance of regular exercise and rest forms the rhythmic dance that keeps the body in harmony.

d. **Emotional Well-Being: The Soul of Fertility**

Emotional well-being is the soul of fertility. Reducing stress, nurturing emotional resilience, and embracing a positive outlook create a fertile ground for conception. Stress management, relaxation techniques, and emotional support are all essential elements of this holistic journey.

e. **Mind-Body Connection: The Power of Positivity**

The mind and body are intricately linked. A positive mindset can influence physical health and fertility. Techniques like meditation, mindfulness, and visualization harness the mind's incredible power to support reproductive health.

- **Holistic Therapies: The Complementary Aspects**

Complementary therapies, from acupuncture to herbal remedies, have been embraced by those on the path to parenthood. These therapies align with the holistic approach, enhancing the body's natural healing mechanisms.

a. Social Support: The Circle of Love

Social support, be it from a partner, family, or friends, forms a circle of love that bolsters fertility. A strong support system provides the emotional foundation on which the journey is built.

b. Environmental Considerations: Nurturing the Nest

Our environment, from the air we breathe to the products we use, can influence fertility. Awareness of potential environmental hazards and adopting a lifestyle that minimizes exposure are crucial elements of holistic fertility.

c. Spirituality: The Soulful Connection

For some, spirituality and faith play an essential role. The connection to something greater than oneself can provide solace and guidance on this deeply spiritual journey.

The holistic approach to fertility is a symphony of elements in perfect harmony. It is the understanding that the mind, body, and spirit are not separate but intricately interwoven. It is the recognition that every choice, from the food we eat to the thoughts we cultivate, influences fertility.

The journey to parenthood is a grand tapestry, woven from the threads of love, biology, and the profound wisdom of the holistic approach. It is a celebration of life, an affirmation of the boundless potential within us, and an acknowledgment that the most extraordinary creations start with the nurturing of body, mind, and spirit. In this journey, we honor the wholeness of life and the hope of new beginnings.

- **Managing Stress and Its Role in Fertility**

In the intricate tapestry of fertility, stress is a thread that often weaves its way into the lives of individuals and couples seeking to conceive. The connection between stress and fertility is a complex one, and managing stress is a pivotal factor in this journey. Let's delve into the profound role that stress plays in fertility and explore the strategies for effective stress management.

A. The Stress-Fertility Connection:

Stress, often regarded as the body's natural response to challenging situations, can be a double-edged sword when it comes to fertility. Elevated stress levels trigger the release of hormones like cortisol and adrenaline, which, when chronic, can disrupt the delicate balance of reproductive hormones.

This disruption can impact fertility in several ways:

Ovulation: Stress may lead to irregular menstrual cycles or even anovulation, hindering the release of eggs necessary for conception.

Implantation: High stress levels can potentially impede the implantation of a fertilized embryo in the uterus.

Miscarriage Risk: Chronic stress may increase the risk of miscarriage

B. **Strategies for Effective Stress Management:** Managing stress is not only beneficial for one's overall well-being but also for enhancing fertility prospects. Here are some powerful strategies to navigate the stress-fertility nexus:

a. *Mindfulness and Relaxation*: Techniques like meditation, deep breathing, and progressive muscle relaxation can help lower stress levels and restore hormonal balance.

b. *Exercise*: Regular physical activity can boost endorphins, reduce stress hormones, and promote overall health, positively impacting fertility.

c. *Nutrition*: A balanced diet rich in essential nutrients can support both physical and emotional well-being.

d. *Support System*: Lean on family and friends for emotional support, and consider joining support groups or seeking professional counseling when needed.

e. *Time Management*: Effective time management can reduce the feeling of being overwhelmed, thus mitigating stress.

f. *Sleep Hygiene*: Prioritize good sleep practices to ensure adequate rest, which is vital for stress reduction.

g. *Holistic Therapies*: Explore alternative therapies such as acupuncture and yoga, which can promote relaxation and balance.

h. *Limiting Stressors*: Identify and reduce sources of stress in your life, whether they are related to work, relationships, or other factors.

i. *Seeking Professional Help*: If stress becomes unmanageable or if you have concerns about fertility, consider consulting a fertility specialist or therapist.

By understanding the profound role that stress plays in fertility and actively managing it, individuals and couples can embark on this journey with greater resilience and hope. Stress, though an inevitable part of life, need not be an insurmountable obstacle. Instead, it can be a catalyst for positive change, fostering a nurturing environment for the creation of life. In the delicate interplay between body and mind, stress management emerges as a powerful tool to empower the pursuit of parenthood.

8. Mindful Living and Fertility

In the quest for parenthood, where the profound desire to conceive meets the complex web of biology and emotion, the concept of mindful living emerges as a beacon of hope and empowerment. Mindfulness, the practice of being fully present in the moment without judgment, holds transformative potential when integrated into the journey of fertility. It offers a path to not only understanding and nurturing one's own body but also to navigating the intricate relationship between stress, emotions, and the ability to conceive.

At its core, mindful living cultivates awareness, acceptance, and compassion for oneself. It encourages individuals and couples to pay close attention to their physical and emotional well-being, to connect with their bodies, and to understand the subtle interplay of thoughts, feelings, and physical health.

- **The Role of Mindfulness in Fertility:**

Mindfulness and fertility intersect on multiple levels:

a. **Stress Reduction**: Mindfulness techniques, such as meditation and deep breathing, are potent tools for managing stress, a known factor in infertility. By reducing the production of stress hormones like cortisol, mindfulness can restore hormonal balance and promote fertility.
b. **Emotional Resilience**: The emotional rollercoaster that often accompanies fertility struggles can be alleviated through mindfulness. It helps individuals acknowledge and process their emotions, fostering resilience and emotional well-being.
c. **Improved Decision-Making**: Mindful living encourages thoughtful decision-making, from choosing a balanced diet to making informed choices about fertility treatments.

d. **Partner Connection**: Mindfulness can enhance communication and connection between partners, fostering a supportive environment in which both can navigate the challenges of infertility together.
e. **Body Awareness**: It promotes a deeper connection with one's body, enabling a better understanding of the menstrual cycle, ovulation, and other critical aspects of fertility.

Practical Applications of Mindful Living in Fertility:

Mindful Meditation: Daily meditation sessions can help individuals remain calm, focused, and present during their fertility journey.

Mindful Eating: Paying attention to what and how you eat can lead to a healthier diet that supports fertility.

Journaling: Keeping a fertility journal allows individuals to track their emotions, physical symptoms, and cycle details mindfully.

Mindful Breathing: Quick mindfulness exercises can be used to manage anxiety and stress during medical procedures or when awaiting pregnancy test results.

In essence, the marriage of mindful living and fertility offers a transformative approach to this deeply personal and often challenging path. It's an invitation to reframe the narrative, replacing anxiety with acceptance, uncertainty with resilience, and isolation with community. Through mindfulness, individuals and couples can navigate the intricacies of fertility with grace, fostering not just the potential for life but also a profound connection with their own inner selves.

- **The Art of Being Present**

In the realm of fertility, where dreams of parenthood meet the challenges of biology, there exists an art, a profound practice that can transform the way one navigates this deeply personal journey. It is the art of being present, a skill that enables individuals and couples to embrace their fertility voyage with authenticity, resilience, and a sense of peace.

a. **The Power of Presence:** Being present means living in the moment, fully immersing oneself in the experiences and emotions of the present, without being weighed down by the past or overwhelmed by the future. In the context of fertility, this practice holds remarkable significance.

b. **Embracing Emotions:** Fertility journeys often come with a rollercoaster of emotions - hope, disappointment, anxiety, and joy. Being present allows individuals to acknowledge and process these feelings, fostering emotional resilience and well-being.

c. **Mind-Body Connection:** The art of being present encourages individuals to connect with their bodies, understanding their menstrual cycles, ovulation, and other crucial aspects of fertility more deeply. This awareness can be empowering and informative.

d. **Reducing Stress:** Living in the present moment naturally reduces stress and anxiety, two factors that can adversely affect fertility. Stress hormones can disrupt hormonal balance and impede conception.

e. **Improving Relationships:** By being fully present with their partners, individuals can strengthen their relationships and build a supportive foundation for the fertility journey. Effective communication, empathy, and connection are nurtured through the art of presence.

Practical Applications of Being Present:
Mindful Breathing: Simple mindful breathing exercises can be practiced daily to stay centered and alleviate stress.

Meditation: Meditation encourages presence and helps individuals remain calm and focused during fertility treatments and the emotional ups and downs of the journey.

Journaling: Keeping a fertility journal is an excellent way to document thoughts and emotions, fostering self-awareness and being present with one's feelings.

The Journey of Resilience: The art of being present is a journey of resilience. It allows individuals to navigate the uncertainties of fertility with grace and strength. Each step, whether it leads to conception or not, becomes a part of a broader narrative, a story of self-discovery, perseverance, and courage.

In a world filled with schedules, expectations, and deadlines, the art of being present offers a sanctuary for authenticity. It's an opportunity to be kind to oneself, to pause and reflect, and to approach the fertility journey with a sense of purpose. It's a reminder that while the destination is parenthood, the true treasures are found in the moments along the way. So, in the midst of hopes and challenges, embrace the art of being present, and let it guide you on this remarkable path to parenthood.

CHAPTER FIVE
Fertility Across Life Stages

9. Fertility From Adolescence to Menopause:
Fertility is not a static chapter in a person's life but a dynamic and evolving journey that spans from adolescence to menopause. This journey reflects the intricate interplay of biology, emotions, and societal expectations, all of which shape an individual's reproductive story.

In essence, the journey of fertility is a lifelong narrative, an intricate tapestry of biology and the human experience. It is not defined by a single phase, but rather by the choices, challenges, and experiences that accompany each stage. From adolescence to menopause, the journey is marked by both the joys of parenthood and the wisdom of self-discovery, reminding us that fertility is not merely about having children but also about embracing life's transitions and choices with grace and resilience.

- **Nurturing Fertility in the Teens: A Delicate Balancing Act**

Fertility is a remarkable gift, a potential that blossoms with puberty, but its care and nurture begin long before most individuals consider parenthood. Nurturing fertility in the teenage years is a vital aspect of reproductive health, as it lays the foundation for a future journey that may lead to parenthood. Here are some essential considerations for promoting fertility in adolescents:

a. Education and Awareness:
Comprehensive sex education: Adolescents should be provided with accurate and age-appropriate sex education that covers not only the basics of reproduction but also topics like contraception, sexually transmitted infections (STIs), and consent.

Understanding the menstrual cycle: Education about the menstrual cycle, ovulation, and the importance of regular periods is crucial to demystify the reproductive process.

b. **Nutrition and Physical Health:** *Balanced diet*: Encourage a diet rich in essential nutrients, including folic acid, iron, and calcium, to support reproductive health. *Physical activity:* Promote regular exercise, as it helps maintain a healthy body weight and regulates hormonal balance.

c. **Mental and Emotional Well-being**: *Stress management:* Adolescents should learn stress-reduction techniques like mindfulness, meditation, and relaxation exercises to safeguard their mental health, as chronic stress can impact reproductive hormones.
   Encourage open communication: Create a safe and open environment for adolescents to discuss their feelings and concerns about their reproductive health.

d. **Safe Sex and Contraception**: **Condom use and contraception**: Adolescents should be educated about the importance of using condoms to prevent STIs and unintended pregnancies. Access to contraception should be readily available and destigmatized.

e. **Avoidance of Harmful Substances**: *Smoking and substance abuse*: Discourage the use of tobacco, alcohol, and recreational drugs, as they can negatively impact reproductive health. *Limit exposure to environmental toxins:* Educate adolescents about the potential risks of exposure to harmful environmental toxins, such as BPA, which may affect fertility.

f. **Regular Health Check-ups:** Encourage routine health check-ups, including gynecological examinations for young women, to ensure reproductive health and detect any potential issues early.

g. **HPV Vaccination:** Recommend the human papillomavirus (HPV) vaccine, which can protect against certain types of HPV that can lead to cervical cancer and impact fertility in the future.

h. Building a Support System: Adolescents should be encouraged to seek support from trusted adults, such as parents, teachers, or healthcare professionals, when they have questions or concerns about their reproductive health.

In nurturing fertility in the teenage years, it's essential to strike a balance between education, empowerment, and support. Adolescents need accurate information, guidance, and a supportive environment to make informed choices about their reproductive health. By focusing on these aspects, we not only empower the next generation with knowledge but also provide them with the tools to protect and nurture their fertility, ensuring a healthier and informed start to their reproductive journey.

- **Fertility Considerations in Midlife**

Midlife is a phase of life marked by transformation and self-discovery, and for many, it's a period where fertility considerations take center stage once again. Understanding fertility in midlife is essential, as it can lead to thoughtful choices and informed decisions regarding family planning. Here are key considerations for individuals and couples entering this transformative stage:

a. Changing Fertility Dynamics: *Fertility Decline:* Midlife, often characterized as the late thirties and forties, brings a natural decline in fertility for both men and women. Women experience a decrease in the number and quality of eggs, making conception more challenging. Men may also notice a gradual decline in sperm quality.

b. Emotional Complexities: *Coping with Challenges:* Fertility issues during midlife can evoke complex emotions, including feelings of frustration, disappointment, and even grief. Recognizing and addressing these emotions is essential for emotional well-being. *Exploring Alternatives*: For those experiencing difficulties, it's a time to explore alternatives such as assisted reproductive technologies (ART) like in vitro fertilization (IVF) or considering adoption or surrogacy.

c. **Health and Lifestyle Choices**: *Self-Care*: Midlife is a period where self-care becomes paramount. Maintaining a healthy lifestyle, which includes a balanced diet, regular exercise, and stress management, can positively impact both overall health and fertility.
Health Check-ups: Regular medical check-ups, particularly gynecological exams for women and fertility evaluations for men, are important.

d. **Assisted Reproductive Technologies (ART)**:
Fertility Treatments: Midlife may be the time when some individuals or couples choose to explore fertility treatments like IVF. The success rates vary, but it can be a viable option. *Egg and Sperm Freezing*: For those who want to preserve their fertility potential, egg and sperm freezing can be considered earlier in life, offering the possibility of using frozen gametes for future family planning.

e. **Emotional Support and Communication:**   *Partnerships*: Open and honest communication with one's partner is essential during this phase. Fertility challenges can affect both individuals, and mutual support is crucial. *Support Systems*: Seeking support from friends, family, or infertility support groups can provide a safe space to share experiences and emotions.

f. **Embracing Diverse Paths**: Understanding that fertility doesn't define one's worth or identity is key. Embracing diverse paths to parenthood, including adoption or surrogacy, offers alternative routes to building a family.

g. **Reflection and Resilience**: Midlife is a time for reflection, self-discovery, and resilience. It's about embracing the possibilities life offers, whether they lead to biological parenthood or alternative routes to building a family.

In conclusion, fertility considerations in midlife present a unique journey filled with challenges and opportunities. It's a time to understand and respect the changes the body undergoes, emotionally adapt to the challenges, and explore the options available. It's also a phase that celebrates resilience, self-care, and the wisdom that comes from navigating this profound transition. Ultimately, midlife fertility considerations are a chapter in the larger story of life, where choices and experiences shape a fulfilling narrative.

- **Menopause: A Journey of Transformation**

Menopause, a phase of life that every woman eventually navigates, is a remarkable journey of transformation. It's a natural biological process that typically occurs in the late 40s or early 50s, marking the end of a woman's reproductive years. While menopause brings physical and hormonal changes, it's also a period of self-discovery, empowerment, and embracing new beginnings.

a. **Physical Changes**

Menopause is characterized by the cessation of monthly menstrual cycles, a result of declining estrogen levels. This change can bring symptoms like hot flashes, night sweats, and changes in sleep patterns. It's important to acknowledge and address these physical changes through medical advice, lifestyle adjustments, and self-care.

b. **Emotional Evolution**

Menopause is not just about the body; it's about the mind and spirit. Women may experience emotional fluctuations, from mood swings to feelings of liberation. It's a time to explore the full range of emotions and prioritize mental well-being.

c. **Empowerment and Freedom**

Menopause liberates women from the worries of contraception and monthly periods. It's an opportunity to rediscover oneself, prioritize personal growth, and pursue passions that may have taken a backseat during the child-rearing years.

d. Wisdom and Experience

With age comes wisdom, and menopause is a time to reflect on life's experiences and lessons. It's an affirmation of resilience, a reminder that each wrinkle and gray hair signifies a unique journey filled with achievements and adventures.

e. Self-Care and Health

Menopause emphasizes the importance of self-care and maintaining good health. It's a stage when women should focus on a balanced diet, regular exercise, and routine health check-ups to ensure overall well-being.

f. Community and Support

Connecting with other women going through menopause can provide a sense of community and support. Sharing experiences and advice can make the journey more manageable and less isolating.

g. New Beginnings

Menopause is not an end but a beginning. It's the start of a life chapter free from the constraints of fertility, offering the chance to pursue personal goals, engage in creative endeavors, and embrace new adventures.

In conclusion, menopause is a multifaceted journey that symbolizes the beauty of aging and personal evolution. It's a celebration of a woman's strength, resilience, and the wisdom that comes with age. Embracing menopause is not about fading away but stepping into a new, empowered, and liberating phase of life. It's a transformation to be celebrated and embraced with open arms.

10. Addressing Fertility Hurdles

The journey to parenthood is a profound aspiration for many, but it's not always a straightforward path. Fertility hurdles can challenge this dream, testing one's resilience, patience, and determination. This journey is marked by complexity, medical decisions, and emotional ups and downs. Addressing fertility hurdles involves a blend of science, emotional strength, and hope. It's a journey that showcases the unwavering human spirit and the pursuit of a dream that transcends obstacles. In this pursuit, we explore the means to navigate these hurdles with grace and perseverance, in the quest to create life and write a beautiful new chapter.

- **Common Fertility Challenges**

The journey to parenthood is often envisioned as a straightforward path, but for many, it's a road marked by common fertility challenges. These obstacles can test one's resolve, patience, and determination, transforming the dream of having a child into a resilient pursuit. Let's explore some of the common fertility challenges couples may encounter:

A. **Irregular Menstrual Cycles:** Irregular periods can make it difficult to predict ovulation, which is a crucial factor in conception. This issue may be linked to conditions such as polycystic ovary syndrome (PCOS) or hormonal imbalances.

B. **Age-Related Decline**: As women age, the quantity and quality of their eggs diminish. This age-related fertility decline often leads to challenges in getting pregnant, particularly after the age of 35.

C. **Male Infertility:** Fertility issues are not limited to women. Male infertility, characterized by low sperm count or reduced sperm motility, can be a significant factor in conception difficulties.

D. **Tubal Blockages**: Blocked or damaged fallopian tubes can impede the journey of an egg to the uterus, making it challenging for fertilization to occur naturally.

E. **Endometriosis**: This condition, where tissue similar to the uterine lining grows outside the uterus, can cause inflammation and scarring, potentially affecting fertility.

F. **Unexplained Infertility:** In some cases, despite extensive testing, the exact cause of infertility remains unknown, making the journey even more frustrating.

G. **Lifestyle Factors**: Habits such as smoking, excessive alcohol consumption, obesity, and high levels of stress can negatively impact fertility.

H. **Polyps or Fibroids**: Growth of polyps or fibroids in the uterus can interfere with implantation or fertility.

I. **Egg Quality**: The quality of a woman's eggs can affect fertility. Certain medical conditions or lifestyle factors can influence egg quality.

J. **Emotional Toll**: Dealing with fertility challenges can be emotionally draining. It often involves a rollercoaster of hope, disappointment, and resilience, affecting the emotional well-being of individuals and couples.

As daunting as these challenges may be, they're not insurmountable. Advancements in medical science, assisted reproductive technologies, lifestyle changes, and emotional support can help address these hurdles. The journey to parenthood often showcases the strength and resilience of those facing these challenges, reinforcing the belief that the pursuit of creating a family is a testament to the unwavering human spirit. It's a journey marked by both obstacles and the determination to overcome them, resulting in the creation of precious life and the fulfillment of a lifelong dream.

- **Strategies for Overcoming Obstacles: Empowering the Journey to Parenthood**

Fertility obstacles can present significant challenges to women on their path to parenthood. These obstacles, whether due to medical conditions or age-related factors, may seem like formidable barriers. However, with determination and the right strategies, women can navigate these hurdles and increase their chances of conceiving. Here are some empowering strategies for overcoming female fertility obstacles:

a. **Seek Professional Guidance:** Consulting a fertility specialist is often the first step. A thorough evaluation can help identify the specific fertility challenges you face, whether they involve irregular periods, hormone imbalances, endometriosis, or other issues.

b. **Hormone Therapy** For some fertility challenges related to hormonal imbalances, hormone therapy may be recommended. This can help regulate the menstrual cycle and improve ovulation.

c. **Surgical Interventions**: In cases where conditions like fibroids or polyps are affecting fertility, surgical procedures can be performed to remove or treat these growths.

d. **Assisted Reproductive Technologies (ART):** For more complex fertility issues, ART options such as in vitro fertilization (IVF), intrauterine insemination (IUI), or egg freezing may be considered. These treatments can increase the likelihood of successful conception.

e. **Egg Donation:** If egg quality is a concern, using donor eggs is a viable option. It can provide a path to parenthood when a woman's own eggs are no longer viable.

f. **Mind-Body Practices:** Incorporating practices like meditation, yoga, and mindfulness can reduce stress and promote relaxation, which can have a positive impact on fertility.

g. **Explore Alternative Paths:** For some, the pursuit of parenthood may take alternative routes, such as adoption or surrogacy. These options offer the possibility of building a family when natural conception is not feasible.

h. **Advocacy and Education:** Being well-informed and an advocate for your own fertility journey is essential. Understanding your options and being an active participant in the decision-making process empowers you to make choices that align with your goals.

Overcoming female fertility obstacles is a journey that demands both physical and emotional resilience. It's a testament to the determination and strength of women who refuse to be defined by these challenges. While the path may be challenging, it also represents an opportunity for personal growth, self-discovery, and the fulfillment of the dream of parenthood. Through informed decisions and support, many women can navigate these obstacles and find success on their unique journey to motherhood.

CHAPTER SIX

Navigating Fertility Treatments

11. Understanding Assisted Reproductive Technologies

Assisted Reproductive Technologies (ART) represent a remarkable intersection of science, hope, and the profound human desire to build a family. This innovative field of medicine has revolutionized the way individuals and couples can overcome fertility challenges and realize their dream of parenthood.

ART encompasses a wide array of advanced techniques, from in vitro fertilization (IVF) to intracytoplasmic sperm injection (ICSI) and beyond. These technologies have not only opened new possibilities for those struggling with infertility but have also redefined the narrative of what it means to become a parent.

In this exploration of ART, we will delve into the intricacies of these cutting-edge methods, shedding light on how they work, their potential benefits, and the emotional journey they entail. Beyond the science, we will uncover the stories of hope, resilience, and the unyielding spirit that accompany those who embark on this path.

The world of ART is a testament to the remarkable progress of medical science and the enduring human spirit. It's a world where the impossible becomes achievable, where the science of conception meets the profound desire for a family. Whether you're considering ART, supporting a loved one, or simply curious about the future of fertility, this journey will be a profound exploration of the awe-inspiring realm of Assisted Reproductive Technologies.

- **An Overview of ART Options**

The journey to parenthood can be a complex and deeply personal one. For some, this path presents unexpected challenges, such as infertility or reproductive health issues. Fortunately, advancements in medical science have given rise to a myriad of Assisted Reproductive Technologies (ART), offering individuals and couples the possibility to overcome fertility obstacles and fulfill their dream of having a child. In this comprehensive overview, we will explore the diverse landscape of ART options, delving into the science, methodologies, and emotional aspects that shape this remarkable journey.

a. **In Vitro Fertilization (IVF):**

The IVF Process: Understand the step-by-step process of IVF, where eggs and sperm are combined outside the body to form embryos.

Indications for IVF: Explore the various situations and conditions for which IVF may be recommended.

IVF Success Rates: Learn about the factors influencing the success of IVF treatments and what to expect throughout the process.

b. **Intracytoplasmic Sperm Injection (ICSI):**

Precision in Fertilization: Discover how ICSI, a technique that involves the injection of a single sperm into an egg, can address male infertility.

Enhancing Fertilization: Learn about the role of ICSI in improving fertilization rates in specific cases.

c. **Donor Eggs and Sperm**:

Donor Eggs: Explore the concept of using donor eggs as a solution to certain fertility challenges.

Donor Sperm: Understand the importance of donor sperm and its role in fertility treatment.

d. **Surrogacy and Gestational Carriers**:

Surrogacy Defined: Discover the concept of surrogacy, where a woman carries and gives birth to a child for another individual or couple.

Gestational Carriers: Learn about the unique role of gestational carriers, women who carry a child biologically unrelated to them.

e. **Cryopreservation Techniques**:

Egg Freezing: Explore the process of freezing and storing a woman's eggs for future use, offering reproductive autonomy and options.

Sperm and Embryo Freezing: Understand the role of freezing sperm and embryos in preserving fertility and supporting ART.

f. Preimplantation Genetic Testing (PGT):

Comprehensive Genetic Screening: Delve into the world of PGT and how it is used to screen embryos for genetic abnormalities.

Impact on Fertility Decisions: Understand how PGT can influence decisions regarding embryo selection during ART treatments.

g. Addressing Male Fertility Challenges:

Male Factor Infertility: Identify the causes of male infertility and the ART options available to overcome them.

Empowering Men in the Fertility Journey: Highlight the role of men in the ART process and their contribution to successful treatments.

h. The Emotional Journey of ART:

Navigating Emotional Complexities: Address the emotional ups and downs associated with fertility treatments and strategies for coping.

Finding Support: Recognize the importance of a strong support system and seek guidance on how to navigate the emotional challenges of the ART journey.

i. Legal and Ethical Considerations:

The Legal Framework: Explore the legal aspects of ART, including regulations, contracts, and parental rights.

Ethical Questions and Debates: Engage in discussions around the ethical considerations and debates within the field of ART.

j. **The ART Success Stories**:

Real-life Triumphs: Share in the inspirational journeys of those who have successfully overcome fertility challenges through ART.

Resilience and Hope: Witness stories of resilience, determination, and the unwavering spirit of individuals and couples in their quest for parenthood.

k. **The Future of Fertility**:

Advances and Innovations: Peer into the future of fertility as we explore the latest advancements and innovations in ART.

Exploring Possibilities: Consider the possibilities that lie ahead for the field, including groundbreaking technologies and emerging trends.

Empowerment Through Knowledge: Understand the power of knowledge in navigating the path to parenthood.

Embracing the Path: Reflect on the journey you are about to embark upon or continue, armed with information, support, and a renewed sense of hope.

"An Overview of ART Options" is your comprehensive guide to understanding the world of Assisted Reproductive Technologies. It is a testament to the remarkable progress of medical science, the enduring human spirit, and the boundless hope that accompanies the pursuit of parenthood. Whether you are at the beginning of your fertility journey, seeking to support a loved one, or simply interested in deepening your knowledge of this extraordinary field, this book will serve as a trusted companion on the path to parenthood.

- **Making Informed Choices**

The decision to explore Assisted Reproductive Technologies (ART) is a pivotal moment on your path to parenthood. It represents an opportunity to overcome fertility challenges and fulfill your dream of having a child. However, making informed choices regarding ART is paramount to ensuring a successful and emotionally fulfilling journey. Here are essential considerations to empower your decision-making process:

a. Seek Expert Guidance:

Consult a Fertility Specialist: Begin your journey by seeking guidance from a qualified reproductive specialist. They can assess your specific situation and recommend the most appropriate ART options.

b. Understand the ART Options:

In-Depth Research: Take the time to thoroughly research the different ART techniques, including IVF, ICSI, donor gametes, surrogacy, and more. Understand the procedures, success rates, and potential risks associated with each.

c. Assess Your Unique Situation:

Personalized Approach: ART should be tailored to your individual needs. Consider factors such as age, overall health, the underlying cause of infertility, and emotional readiness when making decisions.

d. Emotional Preparedness:

Acknowledge the Emotional Journey: Recognize that the ART process can be emotionally taxing. Be prepared for highs and lows, and consider seeking counseling or support to navigate the emotional complexities.

e. Legal and Ethical Considerations:

Know the Legal Framework: Understand the legal aspects of ART, including contracts, parental rights, and any specific regulations in your area.

Ethical Values: Reflect on your ethical beliefs and how they align with the ART choices you make. Address any ethical concerns or dilemmas.

f. Financial Planning:

Cost Considerations: Be aware of the financial aspects of ART. It's crucial to have a clear understanding of the expenses involved and how you plan to manage them.

g. Realistic Expectations:

Success Rates: ART success rates can vary. Maintain realistic expectations about the outcomes of your chosen procedure. Remember that multiple cycles may be necessary for success.

h. Lifestyle Modifications:

Optimize Your Health: Prioritize a healthy lifestyle with a balanced diet, regular exercise, and stress management. These factors can significantly impact the success of ART.

i. Support System:

Build a Network: Create a strong support system of family, friends, or support groups who can offer emotional assistance throughout your ART journey

j. Second Opinions:

Seek Alternative Perspectives: Don't hesitate to seek second opinions from different specialists. Gathering multiple perspectives can provide a well-rounded view of your options.

k. Explore All Paths

Be Open-Minded: While ART is a powerful tool, consider alternative paths to parenthood, such as adoption or surrogacy, if ART does not align with your goals or circumstances.

l. **Empowerment through Knowledge:**
Informed Decision-Making: The more you know about your options, the more empowered you become in making decisions that align with your values and goals.

In conclusion, making informed choices regarding ART is a vital step in your fertility journey. It's a journey marked by hope, science, and a profound desire for parenthood. By seeking expert guidance, understanding your unique situation, and being prepared for the emotional and financial aspects, you can make decisions that empower your path to parenthood. Ultimately, it's about making choices that reflect your values, your hopes, and your determination to create the family you've envisioned.

12. Integrating Nutrition with Fertility Treatments

Nutrition plays a crucial role in optimizing your chances of success during fertility treatments. Whether you're undergoing in vitro fertilization (IVF), intrauterine insemination (IUI), or other ART procedures, a well-balanced diet can be a powerful ally in enhancing fertility. Here's how you can integrate nutrition into your fertility journey:

a. **Prioritize a Balanced Diet:** Consume a variety of nutrient-rich foods, including fruits, vegetables, lean proteins, whole grains, and healthy fats. A balanced diet supports overall health and reproductive function.

b. **Essential Micronutrients**: Pay attention to specific nutrients like folic acid, iron, and vitamin D, which are essential for fertility. You can obtain these through food sources or supplements as recommended by your healthcare provider.

c. **Maintain a Healthy Weight:** Achieving and maintaining a healthy weight can positively impact fertility. Both overweight and underweight conditions can affect hormone balance and ovulation.

d. **Hydration Matters**: Staying well-hydrated is key for overall health and fertility. Water supports bodily functions and helps maintain cervical mucus, which can aid sperm transport.

e. **Antioxidant-Rich Foods**: Antioxidants, found in foods like berries, nuts, and leafy greens, can help protect the eggs and sperm from oxidative stress, potentially improving their quality.

f. **Fertility-Boosting Nutrients:** Certain nutrients like omega-3 fatty acids, found in fish and flaxseeds, have been linked to improved fertility. Incorporate these into your diet.

g. **Limit Processed Foods:** Highly processed foods and excessive sugar intake can lead to inflammation and hormonal imbalances. Minimize these in your diet.

h. **Manage Stress Through Diet:** Foods rich in magnesium, such as leafy greens and nuts, can help manage stress, which is a common component of fertility challenges.

i. **Individualized Nutrition Plans**: Consider consulting a nutritionist who can tailor a diet plan to your specific needs and underlying fertility concerns.

Integrating nutrition with fertility treatments is about nourishing your body to create the optimal environment for conception and a healthy pregnancy. A balanced and mindful approach to eating can enhance your well-being and support your journey to parenthood.

- **Enhancing Treatment Outcomes with Nutrition: Fueling the Path to Fertility Success**

The journey to fertility treatments is a profound and often emotional one. Whether you're embarking on in vitro fertilization (IVF), intrauterine insemination (IUI), or any assisted reproductive technology (ART), optimizing your chances of success is a shared goal. One powerful, yet often underestimated, tool in this quest is nutrition.

Nutrition, as an integral component of overall health, can significantly impact the outcomes of fertility treatments. It provides the essential building blocks for reproductive function, hormonal balance, and the development of healthy eggs and sperm. Here's how you can harness the power of nutrition to enhance your treatment outcomes:

a. **Nourishing Your Reproductive System**: A well-balanced diet rich in fruits, vegetables, whole grains, lean proteins, and healthy fats provides the necessary nutrients to support reproductive health.

b. **Optimizing Egg and Sperm Quality:** Antioxidant-rich foods, such as berries and nuts, help protect eggs and sperm from oxidative damage, potentially improving their quality.

c. **Hormonal Balance:** Certain nutrients, like iron, vitamin D, and omega-3 fatty acids, play a role in hormone regulation. Achieving and maintaining hormonal balance can positively affect fertility.

d. **Weight Management:** Maintaining a healthy weight is essential for fertility. Both excess weight and being underweight can disrupt hormonal balance and ovulation.

e. **Hydration**: Staying well-hydrated supports overall bodily functions and can help maintain cervical mucus, which is crucial for sperm transport.

f. **Stress Reduction:** Foods rich in magnesium and B vitamins, such as leafy greens and nuts, can help manage stress, reducing its impact on fertility.

g. **Individualized Nutrition Plans**: Consider working with a nutritionist who can create a personalized diet plan that aligns with your specific needs and underlying fertility concerns.

h. **Preconception Nutrition:** Preparing your body for treatment through a preconception nutrition plan can optimize your chances of success.

i. **Ongoing Support:**Nutritional support should not be limited to the duration of treatment. Continuously nurturing your body with a balanced diet can help support a healthy pregnancy and post-treatment well-being.

In conclusion, enhancing treatment outcomes with nutrition is about nurturing your body to create the ideal conditions for fertility success. Your diet can be a potent ally on your journey, complementing the expertise of your healthcare providers and the emotional strength you bring to the process. As you embark on this path, remember that each bite you take is a step toward nurturing your fertility and realizing your dream of parenthood.

- **Personalizing Nutrition Plans**

Nutrition is a deeply personal aspect of our lives, intricately linked to our health, well-being, and even our fertility. When it comes to personalizing nutrition plans, there is no one-size-fits-all approach. Instead, it's about crafting a dietary strategy that aligns with your unique needs, goals, and circumstances.

a. **Assessing Your Health and Goals**: Begin by assessing your current health status, including any underlying medical conditions, dietary preferences, and your specific health and wellness goals.

b. **Consulting a Nutrition Professional**: A registered dietitian or nutritionist can be your most valuable ally in personalizing your nutrition plan. They can conduct a comprehensive evaluation and provide expert guidance.

c. **Identifying Nutritional Deficiencies:** Understand any potential nutrient deficiencies in your diet. This can include vitamins, minerals, or macronutrients that may need special attention.

d. **Dietary Preferences and Restrictions**: Take into account your dietary preferences, whether you're vegetarian, vegan, or have food allergies. Your nutrition plan should align with your eating style.

e. **Hormonal Balance and Fertility Goals**: If you're on a fertility journey, consider how your nutrition plan can support hormonal balance and optimize your fertility goals.

f. **Weight Management:** Whether you aim to lose, gain, or maintain weight, your nutrition plan can be tailored to meet your specific weight management goals.

g. **Lifestyle and Activity Level**: Factor in your activity level and lifestyle. An athlete's nutrition plan will differ from that of a sedentary individual.

h. **Mindful Eating**: Incorporate principles of mindful eating, focusing on the quality of your food, portion control, and being in tune with your body's hunger and fullness cues.

i. **Monitoring Progress**: Regularly review and adjust your nutrition plan as needed. Track your progress towards your goals and make modifications as you go along.

j. **Emotional and Psychological Factors:** Recognize that emotional and psychological factors can impact your dietary choices. Address stress, emotional eating, and other psychological components of nutrition.

k. **Long-Term Sustainability**: Your nutrition plan should be sustainable in the long run. It's not about temporary diets but establishing a healthy, lifelong approach to eating.
l. **Regular Check-Ins**: Schedule periodic check-ins with your nutrition professional to ensure your nutrition plan continues to meet your evolving needs.

Personalizing nutrition plans is a journey of self-discovery and well-being. It's about embracing the uniqueness of your body, preferences, and goals. By crafting a nutrition plan that aligns with your individuality, you can optimize your health, support your fertility journey, and foster a lifelong relationship with nourishing your body. Remember that you are your best advocate when it comes to your health and wellness.

CHAPTER SEVEN
Preparing for Pregnancy and Beyond

13. Preconception Nutrition and Health: Cultivating the Foundation of New Life

Before the first ultrasound captures the flutter of a tiny heart or the first cry of a newborn fills the air, there exists a profound phase that shapes the journey of parenthood. This is the period of preconception, where potential parents embark on a transformative path to prepare their bodies, minds, and spirits for the creation of new life. Preconception nutrition and health, like seeds carefully sown in fertile soil, are the bedrock upon which the dreams of a family are built.

The Prelude to Parenthood: Preconception is the period leading up to conception. During this phase, prospective parents have the power to influence the health and well-being of their future child.

a. **Nutrition: A Cornerstone of Preconception Health:** A well-balanced diet rich in essential nutrients serves as the foundation of preconception health. Nutrients such as folic acid, iron, calcium, and omega-3 fatty acids are key players in promoting reproductive health.
b. **Fertility and Hormonal Harmony:** Preconception nutrition supports the delicate balance of hormones, ensuring regular menstrual cycles and optimal ovulation. A healthy body weight and appropriate nutrient intake are essential for promoting fertility.
c. **Avoiding Harmful Substances:** The preconception phase necessitates steering clear of harmful substances such as tobacco, excessive alcohol, and recreational drugs. These can impair fertility and pose risks to fetal development.

d. **Chronic Condition Management:** Prospective parents with chronic health conditions like diabetes, hypertension, or thyroid disorders should actively manage these conditions in consultation with healthcare professionals to optimize fertility.

e. **Folate for Neural Tube Health:** Adequate intake of folic acid is of paramount importance during preconception and early pregnancy. This nutrient is a potent safeguard against neural tube defects in the developing fetus.

f. **Lifestyle and Physic**: A physically active lifestyle can boost fertility and overall health. Incorporating regular exercise, stress management techniques, and quality sleep fosters preconception well-being.

g. **Guarding Against Environmental Toxins:** Limiting exposure to environmental toxins and pollutants is essential. These substances can disrupt reproductive health and potentially harm the growing fetus.

h. **Supplementation and Professional Guidance**: In certain cases, healthcare providers may recommend supplements or nutritional counseling to address specific deficiencies or health concerns.

i. **Dental and Mental u**: Prioritizing oral health and effectively managing mental health conditions is integral to a successful preconception phase.

j. **Shared Responsibility**: Preconception health is a shared commitment between both partners. Each must actively engage in nurturing their health and well-being to create an optimal environment for conception.

The Commencement of an Extraordinary Journey: Preconception health is the starting point of an extraordinary journey. It is a phase illuminated by the light of hope, the anticipation of new life, and the profound commitment to cultivate the foundation of a family.

In summation, preconception nutrition and health are the invisible architects of a healthy pregnancy and the well-being of a future child. Choices made during this sacred phase carry the promise of generations to come, embodying the timeless truth that the journey of life begins with care, intention, and love.

- **Building a Strong Foundation for Pregnancy: Nurturing Life's Beginnings**

Pregnancy, a remarkable journey that culminates in the birth of a new life, begins long before the first signs of a baby bump. It commences with the careful preparation of a fertile soil—the body and mind of the expectant mother—to welcome and nurture the seed of life. Building a strong foundation for pregnancy is not just about the physical aspect; it encompasses emotional, nutritional, and lifestyle considerations. Here's how to prepare for this incredible voyage:

a. **Emotional Readiness**: Preparing for pregnancy means not only taking care of your physical health but also your emotional well-being. Ensure you're ready for the emotional demands and joys of parenthood.
b. **Prenatal Counseling**: Consider seeking prenatal counseling or therapy if you have concerns or unresolved emotional issues that may affect your pregnancy journey.
c. **Avoid Harmful Substances:** Eliminate harmful habits such as smoking, excessive alcohol consumption, and illicit drug use to create a healthier environment for your baby's development.
d. **Fertility Awareness:** If you're actively trying to conceive, become familiar with your menstrual cycle and ovulation. Understanding your fertility window is a valuable tool.
e. **Weight Management:** Achieve and maintain a healthy weight, as being overweight or underweight can affect fertility and pregnancy health.
f. **Prenatal Vitamins**: Discuss with your healthcare provider and start taking prenatal vitamins or supplements as recommended. Folic acid is especially important in the early stages of pregnancy.

g. **Mindful Lifestyle**: Mindful living can be profoundly beneficial. Engage in practices like yoga and mindfulness to promote emotional and mental well-being.

building a strong foundation for pregnancy is a holistic endeavor that extends beyond physical health. Emotional readiness, nutrition, lifestyle, and wellness practices all play pivotal roles. This foundation not only ensures a healthier pregnancy but also cultivates the ideal environment for the growth of a new life. It is a nurturing embrace, welcoming the miracle of motherhood.

- **Personalized Preconception Planning**

Personalized preconception planning is about recognizing that no two paths to parenthood are alike and that each one deserves individualized care and attention. It's the art of crafting a roadmap to pregnancy that aligns with your specific needs, aspirations, and circumstances.

The Significance of Preconception Planning: Preconception planning is the vital phase before conception occurs. It offers the opportunity to optimize health, address potential obstacles, and increase the chances of a healthy pregnancy.

a. **Personalized Health Assessment:** Begin your journey with a thorough health assessment. This includes evaluating your medical history, any existing health conditions, and lifestyle factors.
b. **Nutritional Analysis:** Work with a healthcare provider or nutritionist to assess your dietary habits and nutritional intake. Identify areas where your diet may need adjustments to support fertility and pregnancy.
c. **Lifestyle Considerations:** Reflect on your lifestyle choices, including stress management, exercise routines, and exposure to environmental toxins. Personalized planning considers the unique circumstances of your life.

d. **Emotional and Psychological Wellness:** Address emotional and psychological factors that can influence fertility and pregnancy, seeking therapy or counseling when needed.

e. **Family Planning Goals:** Set clear family planning goals. Determine the number of children you desire and the timing of each pregnancy, if possible.

f. **Medication and Supplements**: If you're on any medications or supplements, discuss their safety and necessity during preconception and pregnancy with a healthcare provider.

Personalized preconception planning is the embodiment of the belief that every journey to parenthood is unique and should be honored as such. It is the recognition that your path is distinct, your desires are one-of-a-kind, and your needs deserve personalized attention. By crafting a preconception plan tailored to your individual circumstances, you set the stage for a more intentional and empowered journey to parenthood, guided by your own unique stars.

14. Partner Support for Fertility: *The Pillar of Strength in the Journey to Parenthood*

The path to parenthood is a shared voyage, and partner support is the cornerstone of this extraordinary journey. It's a testament to the strength of love and commitment, where two individuals come together to navigate the challenges and joys of fertility. In this exploration of partner support for fertility, we delve into the critical role that understanding, empathy, and unwavering encouragement play in the pursuit of a common dream: the gift of life.

- **The Role of Partners in the Fertility Journey:** *A Symphony of Support and Understanding*

The journey to parenthood is a profound expedition, marked by hope, longing, and sometimes, unexpected challenges GNB. Within this remarkable voyage, the role of partners in the fertility journey is a symphony of support, understanding, and shared determination. It's a testament to the strength of love and commitment, where two individuals come together to navigate the intricate path to parenthood. In this exploration, we unveil the multifaceted role that partners play in this extraordinary quest.

A. **Emotional Anchors**: Partners serve as emotional anchors, offering unwavering support through the highs and lows of fertility treatments. Their presence provides comfort and assurance, making the journey less daunting.

B. **Shared Dreams and Goals:** Together, partners form a united front, sharing dreams and goals of building a family. Their joint commitment provides a powerful driving force to overcome obstacles.

C. **Fostering Open Communication**: Effective communication is key. Partners who openly discuss their thoughts, feelings, and concerns can better understand each other's needs and provide comfort and solace.

D. **Financial Planning and Decision-Making**: Partners collaborate on important decisions related to fertility treatments, including financial planning. Their joint efforts ensure a clear path forward.

E. **Attending Medical Appointments**: Accompanying each other to medical appointments fosters a sense of togetherness. Partners are often present to lend support, ask questions, and take an active role in the process.

F. **Sharing the Load:** In the physical aspects of fertility treatments, such as administering medications or tracking ovulation, partners share the responsibilities and lighten the load.

G. **Emotional Resilience**: Partners contribute to emotional resilience, acting as sounding boards and sources of strength during the more challenging phases of the journey.

H. **Being Informed and Advocates**: Partners educate themselves about the fertility process and advocate for each other's needs, ensuring a supportive and well-informed partnership.
I. **Celebrating Milestones:** Partners find joy in celebrating milestones, no matter how small, as each step forward is a testament to their shared determination.
J. **Embracing Changes:** Partners adapt to changes and challenges together. They offer empathy and patience as the fertility journey evolves.
K. **Reinforcing Love and Commitment:** The fertility journey can be a profound test of love and commitment. Partners who navigate it together often emerge with their bond strengthened.
L. **Coping with Setbacks:** Partners provide a safe space to grieve and cope with setbacks. Their unwavering support helps in finding hope amidst disappointment.
M. **Respecting Individual Experiences:** Partners recognize that the fertility journey can be a unique experience for each individual. They respect and validate each other's emotions and responses.

The role of partners in the fertility journey is of immense significance. It's a partnership rooted in love, strengthened by shared dreams, and characterized by unwavering support. Together, partners create a harmonious environment that nurtures the hope for new life. It is a testament to the power of unity in the face of challenges and the depth of love in the pursuit of parenthood.

CHAPTER EIGHT

Real Fertility Stories

Real fertility stories are personal accounts that reveal the poignant and often challenging journeys of individuals and couples facing infertility. These narratives provide a candid and unfiltered glimpse into the emotional and physical hurdles that accompany fertility challenges. They serve as powerful reminders that real-life success stories are born out of determination, resilience, and unwavering hope.

15. A Source of Inspiration

Fertility Stories as a Source of Inspiration: Narratives of Triumph and Hope

Fertility stories are powerful and poignant narratives that provide a beacon of hope and inspiration to those navigating the complex and emotional terrain of infertility. They serve as a testament to the human spirit's resilience and the enduring strength of individuals and couples facing fertility challenges. These stories are more than just personal accounts; they are a source of encouragement, support, and a reminder that success is attainable even in the face of adversity.

a. **Breaking the Silence:** Fertility stories often begin with individuals and couples breaking the silence surrounding their struggles. Opening up about their journey can be the first step toward seeking support and finding inspiration.
b. **Triumph Over Adversity:** These stories illustrate the triumph of the human spirit over adversity. They demonstrate that with determination, individuals can overcome the most daunting of obstacles.
c. **Bridging Isolation:** Infertility can be an isolating experience, but fertility stories bridge that gap. They assure those facing similar challenges that they are not alone in their journey.

d. **Providing Information and Awareness:** Fertility stories offer insights into the medical, emotional, and psychological aspects of infertility. They serve as an educational resource for those seeking information.

e. **Encouraging Emotional Healing:** Many fertility stories highlight the emotional healing process. Sharing one's struggles and triumphs can be a therapeutic way to cope with the emotional toll of infertility.

f. **Celebrating Small Victories:** Fertility stories often celebrate the small victories along the way, reminding individuals that each step forward is an achievement to be cherished.

g. **Embracing Diverse Paths to Parenthood**: These stories emphasize that there is no one-size-fits-all solution to infertility. They reveal the various paths to parenthood, including natural conception, assisted reproductive technologies, adoption, and surrogacy.

h. **Offering Hope:** Fertility stories are, at their core, a wellspring of hope. They inspire individuals and couples to continue their journey, even when the path seems uncertain.

i. **Fostering Empathy and Understanding:** Sharing one's experience with infertility fosters empathy and understanding. It encourages a more compassionate and supportive community for those facing similar challenges.

j. **A Testimony of Love and Commitment:** For couples, fertility stories are a testimony to their love and commitment. They illustrate the depth of a partnership and the shared dream of parenthood.

Fertility stories are a source of inspiration, a beacon of hope for those facing the daunting journey of infertility. They are a testament to the strength of the human spirit, the endurance of love, and the unshakable commitment to the dream of parenthood. These stories exemplify that even in the face of adversity, there is always room for hope, and success is a journey that can be achieved through unwavering determination and a supportive community.

CONCLUSION

In closing, **"Nourish to Flourish: The Science of Female Fertility and Nutrition"** has been a journey of discovery and empowerment. We've delved deep into the intricate connection between nutrition and female fertility, uncovering the profound impact it has on the lives of women. As we wrap up this exploration, I want to leave you with a resounding message of hope and possibility.

1. **The Power of Nutrition**: Throughout this book, we've witnessed the incredible influence of nutrition on female fertility. It's become abundantly clear that what we eat directly impacts our reproductive health.

2. **Balanced Diet, Balanced Life:** A balanced and wholesome diet is not just a recipe for fertility; it's a recipe for a vibrant and thriving life. It's the foundation upon which we can build our reproductive wellness.

3. **Understanding Your Body**: One of the key takeaways is the importance of understanding your own body. Women's bodies are unique, and knowing how your body functions is the first step toward optimizing your fertility.

4. **Lifestyle Choices Matter**: It's not only about what's on your plate but also about how you live your life. Managing stress, getting enough sleep, and staying physically active are all integral to the fertility equation.

5. **Nutrient-Rich Foods**: The book has emphasized the role of specific nutrients, from folic acid to antioxidants, in nurturing fertility. Incorporating these foods into your diet can make a substantial difference.

6. **The Role of Hormones**: Hormones play a central role in fertility. By embracing a diet that supports hormonal balance, you can enhance your chances of conceiving and maintaining a healthy pregnancy.

7. **Long-Term Health**: This journey isn't just about conceiving; it's about securing your long-term health. The same principles that improve fertility can also guard against chronic diseases and promote a vibrant, graceful aging process.

8. **Hope and Resilience:** Infertility can be an emotionally challenging journey. "Nourish to Flourish" reminds us that there is always hope, and resilience is your greatest ally.

9.**Empowerment through Knowledge:** Knowledge is power. Armed with the scientific insights shared in this book, you have the tools to take control of your fertility and health.

10. **The Path to Flourishing**: We conclude with the belief that every woman has the potential to flourish. The path may be unique for each of us, but by nourishing our bodies, embracing knowledge, and making informed choices, we can unlock the remarkable potential within us.

Our bodies are incredible ecosystems, finely tuned to respond to the nourishment we provide. The science we've uncovered here proves that with mindful dietary choices, we can enhance our fertility, boost our reproductive health, and ultimately, pave the way for a flourishing future.

Remember that fertility is not just about bearing children; it's about embracing your vitality, understanding your body, and harnessing the incredible potential within you. As women, we are warriors, nurturers, and creators. "Nourish to Flourish" is a testament to our ability to take control of our health and fertility, making informed decisions that can shape the course of our lives.

Let this book be your guiding light, your source of knowledge, and your companion on your journey toward a healthier, more fertile you. Whether you're starting a family, preserving your fertility for the future, or simply seeking optimal well-being, your path to flourishing begins with the nourishment you provide yourself.

May "Nourish to Flourish" inspire you to make the choices that honor your body, embrace your fertility, and allow you to thrive in every aspect of your life. The power to nourish and flourish is within your grasp. It's time to step confidently into the world, knowing that you hold the key to your own vitality and the promise of a future rich with possibilities. Thank you for embarking on this enlightening journey with us, and may your path be filled with health, happiness, and abundance.